UNDERCOVER MIRACLE TEAM

A Christian Novel

Based on True Testimonies

by

Lynne Suszek

ISBN: 9781795222563

Foreword by Pastor Nick Boork

"The "Undercover Miracle Team" is a book that has the effect of making you feel that you're not only observing miracles as they happen before your eyes but that they can happen through you too by acting in faith on the promises of God! Having experienced the power of God flowing through me on several occasions to heal people I am convinced that this book will stir you up to believe God to manifest his miracles through you as well. Lynne Suszek brings us a much needed fresh perspective on the supernatural work that the Holy Spirit is longing to do through those that will step out of the boat and go where they have never walked with Jesus as his Ambassadors no matter where they live as Christ commanded the apostles to go into "all the world and preach the gospel with signs following! May God be glorified as you read and act by faith in Jesus name!"

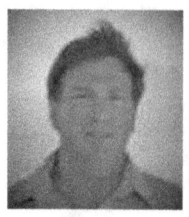 Pastor Nick Boork is author of "Developing the Preacher Within You" available on Amazon, founder of Diamond Institute and Diamond Ministerial Association a Spirit filled group that provides ministerial credentials and ordination. He also is author of the One Year Bible Club covering the entire New Testament with his teaching commentary daily. See more on his website: www.nickboork.com

Pastor Nick ordained Mark and Lynne Suszek into the ministry on Dec 3 2017. View their ordination on Youtube at this link Suszek Ordination or go to TheBibleTek Channel.

https://www.youtube.com/channel/UC9TMbYglqIoS-64coulPlTg

Contents

Chapter 1

Unfamiliar Territory

How he ended up in Africa on a mission trip was a story only written in some books in heaven's library. Joel Phillips was a detective just like he always wanted, yet he hadn't known that it was part of God's plan for him until now. A homicide police officer is used to seeing dead bodies; only in his line of duty, in his own territory, they always stay dead. On a missions trip in Africa, dead bodies aren't staying dead. The team told him that God calls Christians to raise the dead, heal the sick and cast out demons but nothing could really prepare him for it. Maybe he thought he believed, or wanted to believe it could happen but the natural mind cannot comprehend a miracle. It was time to think with his born-again spirit for this to make sense. The man on the ground was dead. He was executed by some gang that no longer had any use for him. In a pool of blood, the team happened upon him and Brandy, the E.R. nurse who was experienced in Detroit Receiving, a very busy hospital with high traffic of emergencies, assessed him to be deceased. The Emergency Medical Tech also agreed that he was as dead as anyone they had ever seen. But this group was on a mission of life and miracles. Some had done this many times and others, never before. One of them shouted in faith, an all-encompassing "Life!" to the body, just as he was trained by his ministry team. Another simply commanded "Sir! Get back into your body and get up, NOW!"   The authoritative voices stirred the atmosphere and fear disappeared - excitement entered the group. Shouts and expectation went on for either a minute or an eternity .. Joel felt it was both. Staring at the corpse, Joel tilted his head and stepped back as the body twitched. A deep breath was taken by the corpse. Coughing, a sneeze and eyes now opening, the stiff, lifeless body became revived! Shouts of relief and screams from the inexperienced were sounding off. "Sir! Jesus has raised you from the dead! We are praying over you!" "Get up!" someone directed him. The black man of about 25 years was shocked but receptive. Blood was dried up on his head and no more fresh was coming. The crowd acted as any emergency room team ever has in helping him but their expectancy of full recovery was higher than any hospital ever gets. Praising and singing filled the air. Joel did whatever he was told in order to help. The man was being told about Jesus and salvation. He nodded and smiled eagerly. Joel had seen a man raised from the dead. How could he go back to his job as usual? How could he ever view death as final again? The missions trip was a successful training ground for miracles, this medical-background team of Christians would never be the same. Learning how it's done supernaturally just ruins the medical, natural mind and the old training just will no longer do!

From a combination of testimonies of raising the dead, one of which was through ministry leader Andrew Wommack. A man was raised by the command "Get back into your body!"

Chapter 2

Back in the States

Back in "The States," Joel promises to meet weekly with his new team. His spiritual and physical worlds are actually now both realities that are in effect, tangible. Telling anyone about the trip feels pointless even at church. Blank stares is all he can expect from anyone other than his team. Raising the dead, healing the sick and yes, absolutely, demons are real so casting out demons is also real. Joel somehow feels the miracles slipping away like a dream though. How can he keep it in his experience on a frequent basis, he asks himself and knows God is listening. It is not that there's stronger faith in other countries making miracles happen, he evaluates. It is only the willingness to use the power available in us (in Christ) that changes as we step outside the comfy-cozy USA, where life is only an emergency once in a while. Africans face war and need miracles often. War zones are 24/7 emergency areas, therefore Christians in war zones are less able to solve matters without miracles. If we don't need miracles we stop expecting them. If we don't know how to expect a miracle, we don't get one. The weekly meetings helped to rekindle the excitement of the missions trip but Joel felt a tug from deep within to keep this going. "Let's see, what opportunities do we have here to raise the dead?" asked a big ominous voice that was very familiar in Joel's mind. The voice was just a warm, profound thought that penetrated his own thoughts with almost a chuckle or a warm smile attached. "Ooooo nooo" Joel thought back.. "you can't be serious!" Joel shouted in his mind. Joel's job as a detective gave him more opportunities with fresh corpses than a mortician. "What can happen if a corpse that has been thoroughly declared dead by a medical examiner gets up and walks away? What can happen if it always happens around me?" Joel thought. "What if it was murder?" The very thought boggled his brain and made his logical mind crawl. SLAP! He wanted someone to wake him up. He wanted to run and hide like Jonah and the whale. "Why me?" Joel asked. As he was chickening out of every thought, a call shook him up and rattled his whole body. It was a call to duty as his captain asked him to come look at a homicide. "We have a body." His captain's voice was calm and emotionless as usual. 30 year old woman strangled, in the park. Joel's automatic professional response gave a chill to his own spine. "I'll be right there." Flash backs of 5 people raised from the dead in Uganda were running through his mind. One of them came back by Joel's own command. He replayed the moment over and over. Visions of each one were running through his memory as if by force. "What's the difference between them and this woman?" came a penetrating thought. He choked on his own answer. "Just the audience." When Joel approached the woman's body, it lay lifeless in an awkward position. Yellow tape surrounded the area. Reporting her ID to Joel, "mother of two children, wife" his associate filled him in. "Thank you " he said and compassion welled up inside him to his throat as if it might speak out of his vocal cords "GET UP!" But Joel stopped it and asked everyone to give him space to examine the area. Not an odd request. So they did. Walking away, they went to fill out reports and leave him to himself. Joel turned around and looked upon the lady.

Compassion welled up again uncontrollably; Joel leaned over to her ear and spoke before his natural mind could win over and draw him back. "Get up!" He said in a small shout. A whisper is just not going to raise the dead. But no one was looking and nobody else prayed with him in support this time. Fighting with his natural mind again he shouted in her ear, "GET UP LADY! YOUR KIDS NEED YOU! GET BACK INTO YOUR BODY IN JESUS' NAME!" Experience from the missions trip had caused his heart to expect a miracle and all the faith he had choked him. "She's not dead" came a penetrating thought, "believe that." Joel touched her arm. She was getting warm. "Oh my God" both excitement and fear rushed in. The Holy Spirit was jumping up and down in him. Fear and doubt tried to steal the show saying

"You're crazy! It's not happening! What will they say?" Joel shook her a little like he was waking someone up. He said her name "Miss Jenny! I mean Mrs!" and then "Breathe!!" he commanded. Like a vacuum suddenly turning on, GASP!! The body breathed! Peace flooded the area and fear was gone. His coworker was running in to see.. "What the… !!!@&$?!!!" Dave cursed. People were gathering around. Joel shouted "give her space!" Dave declared "she was dead!" Joel sharply replied "Not anymore!" Dave could hardly speak "What did you do?? CPR? Witchcraft?"

"Ha! Satan would love to take the credit… no, something I learned on my missions trip.."

"Ma'am! You're back!" She opened her eyes in bewilderment. Her neck had been rope-burned but was quickly healing. The team of emergency medics and officers were standing and staring in amazement. Firemen, EMTs all holding papers but too stunned to speak. The lady got up to her feet and began to cry. "Who strangled you maaam?" Joel sat her on a bench. He covered her with blankets and as detectives do, he questioned her. "Oh my freaking God .. I was strangled!" she recalled the event and went over it. Describing the man and how he attacked her, details were taken down. Joel was ecstatic at the idea of finding the murderer by the eye-witness of the victim herself.

This event was passed off as a misdiagnosed death; strangling is one way that death symptoms are known to be misread. Joel shared this miracle at his next meeting. He was pummeled with questions and praising of God.

"Working in the ER, I don't know what I could do to raise the dead!" Brandy started. "We are monitored all the time and I can't shout WAKE

UP at every corpse… can I?" Silence followed as everyone was equally put in the spotlight. This team was a group of medical professionals who went on a missions trip under a ministry that believes in healing and dead-raising. The Authority of the Believer by Andrew Wommack was one book that they studied and Dominion Life Church is another ministry they all followed as well. Currie Blake in that church had taken the leadership role after John G. Lake, one of the big names who taught on miraculous ministry. Miracles are expected there! Both of these modern-day-Pauls had raised one of their own children from the dead. Their examples are some kind of act to follow eh? Deaf ears opened today, blind eyes see… everything in the book of Acts still happens and more. The apostles are our first examples but living amongst us are people practicing and teaching miracles today.

"I'm sure God wants us to do it." Pastor Mark said. "Not sure how to keep raising the dead without getting bad press and accused of fraud but that's a risk worth taking. If we ask Him, God can show us how to do it so that we can stay put in our jobs and keep on doing it! God's calling is higher than our jobs I think!" Pastor Mark had no experience in what we were dealing with but he was right about the higher calling. Miracles mixed into a profession is not in the Bible. Raising the dead is a concept for which emergency teams have the most opportunity. Hospice nurses, EMTs, detectives and policemen, fire men and emergency room teams have access to those who need immediate miracles. It seemed to this group that God was stirring up a team in the U. S. A. to do secret undercover work for the gospel. He was raising up Emergency Miracle Technicians! A new Team Awesome! If we can't have the dead being brought to the churches for prayer, we need undercover miracle technicians in the hospitals! "But why the secrecy?" Tom challenged, arms folded. "Why not shout and give glory to God? Wouldn't we want it be reported on the news?"

Pastor Mark sighed deeply and looked at his modern-day disciples. "We saw what happened by being bold in the gospels. The envy of the world, the doctors, even pastors would cause trouble for us exactly like the Pharisees in Jesus' day! Darkness is offended by the light. Discreetness is not unscriptural. Jesus was discreet in many cases."

Each one imagined what problems could happen by not being discreet with prayer on-the job.

Chapter 3

On-The-Job Miracles

B randy pondered the thought of miracles on the job. Everyone on the mission trip was so excited to experience raising the dead and healing in that war zone but coming back to the states was like a cold slap in the face. Demonic voices taunted them all "that stuff doesn't happen here; it's only on the special trips!" And again "don't you dare try that here! You'll lose your career! You'll be locked up!" Brandy knew these thoughts were not from God. She knew that Satan was trying to discourage her. "Don't even think about it!" shouted her thoughts. Her heart struggled not to agree with those thoughts. It wasn't long before Brandy would be faced with a decision and she knew which was the right one. "Lord help me to discreetly pray for people on my job." she whispered. On her next shift at the emergency room in Detroit, hardly a day would pass where death was not faced. An asthma victim came in struggling for air. This 10 year old girl was having an attack and she was hyperventilating fast. The little girl turning blue, Brandy took a moment between medical procedures to pray. She leaned over to the girl as if time slowed down and only she and the girl were in the room. It felt like everyone else was in slow motion and a bubble surrounded them. Heaven watched as Brandy spoke into her ear with authority "Fear leave! Wheezing stop! Breathe Emma breathe! In Jesus' Name!"

The wheezing became deep, grateful breaths and as if something let go of her throat, color started returning and a warm glow of peace came over the girl. Emma looked at the nurse with grateful eyes and wonder. She would not forget those words or the nurse who spoke them. Brandy was filled with relief and embarrassment. Shame tried to accuse her and scold her for acting in faith. "This is not a church!" she heard. "What if someone heard you? What if it didn't work? What if the girl tells someone what you did?" Brandy decided she must not let Satan be allowed to go unanswered: she spoke back to the thoughts under her breath "Shut up! Get behind me! Fear of man brings a snare." And the onslaught was silenced. The room was busy and now people were asking Emma how she was feeling. "Are you ok? Here's some oxygen for you" a mask was offered. Emma breathed deeply and kept looking at the nurse. Brandy and

Emma met eyes a few times and the atmosphere was deflating to a non-emergency. Everyone involved had different thoughts about what happened and never asked Brandy what she said to the girl. "Thank you Lord" Brandy closed her eyes and sighed. Embarrassed that it was not hard to do, she thought about why it took her so long to do this? Nevertheless, now is always a good time for miracles. He is a God of "nows."

Actual account taken from an account of Mark Suszek on a canoe trip with a group of 6th graders

Chapter 4

Conviction of What We Have

The miracle team met again. Now Brandy shared what she did on her shift. "It wasn't hard" she confessed. "I knew what to do. I've been trained to speak to the problem and not beg God to do it. I've been practicing my faith for myself and my family with good results for years." The others agreed and all were convicted of their own ability-in-Christ to do the same. "We all have the power that raised Christ from the dead in us." Pastor Mark commented. "What holds us back? Fear of course." he answered himself. Luke, the

Emergency Medical Technician recalled the trip in Uganda. His knowledge as a medical professional was in competition with his faith there. But the group operated as miracle workers so he did too. Luke was just reflecting on how easy it is to operate in faith when you are with a whole group who is using faith for miracles. When on-the-job however, the carnal thinking takes precedence. His five senses are usually in control in medical groups.   Flashbacks of undeniable miracles pierced his conscience. The faces of women, children and elderly came rushing to his remembrance. A leader there showed a whole town the power of God by asking for the deaf to be brought up to her. Deaf people were brought to the front. As a show of God's power she tested their hearing one by one. The town knew they were deaf. "Ears open! In Jesus' Name!" She shouted. Then retested their hearing. The deaf person reacted to her voice and the town was amazed. Salvation was preached and many gave their hearts to Jesus. It's risky business doing something like that. The miracle has to happen or else! Missionaries like that are all-in for the faith poker game. There's no faking it and it must happen immediately not later or slowly. Here in the states, rarely are churches believing for miracles. They don't expect them or know how to pray. Luke also learned like the others in this group, to command heath by speaking to the body like Jesus told lame people "arise!" and called the dead "come forth!" with a loud voice. "Ears open!" "pain go!" "eyes see!" is the effective way to see miracles. Also the method of expectation through thanksgiving "thank you Lord that my husband will live and not die" over and over is effective as taught by Norvel Hayes and others. Another ministry teaches just to speak "life" and believe. Luke decided it was time to start using his faith-authority on the job. His next shift was slow as he watched the clock. A watched pot never boils they say. But finally an emergency came. Ambulance lights on. Siren blaring. 90 miles per hour to the site. Child fell out of a window face down. People crying, the 3 year-old was lifeless. Moving her with careful precision she lay there on a stretcher. CPR was not done due to the facial damage. "Bring her in here!" Luke said pulling her into the ambulance. The unbelief was tangible but Luke closed the door and began speaking life. "Thank you Lord that she will live and not die, thank you Lord that she will live and not die" Luke repeated. The ambulance was on its way to the hospital and Luke was surrounded by a host of angels who harken to the voice of God's Word. Luke felt the peaceful presence of heaven and spoke to the girl, "live!" then the joy of the Lord welled up. Laughter came from deep within his belly and he laughed over her. As inappropriate as it seems to the natural mind, laughter is medicine, the Bible says. So he allowed the laughter out and kept laughing. The driver heard him and was so shocked by it he screamed "what's going on, man!?" Luke was laughing so hard tears rolled down his face. The little girl gasped for air, breathed in like she was thrown back into her body forcefully and began to cry and giggle. Luke spoke to her bones and face to heal quickly. "Teeth and face mend!" Nose you repair!" The driver yelled again, "Jay!!" This time Luke answered, "Ha!! She's back!" The driver said, "who's back? Who are you talking to? Are you ok, man?" Luke answered, "This little girl is back!" "Whoaaaaa! Say what? Are you for real?" the young driver was not able to take it in. Then the crying and giggling sound of a child was louder.

The man driving pulled in to the hospital, parked and ran to the back of the ambulance opening the doors like a Christmas present. The face of the driver was pale even though he was a black man. He stared as if seeing a ghost. Luke was holding the little girl in his arms like a daddy, she looked at the driver with a badly scraped face but teeth were intact and she smiled. "Where's my mommy?" she said. The driver couldn't speak. Luke said "let's go get examined!" and walked into the hospital carrying little Sophie. The parents arrived there in the waiting room crying. When Luke came out to say "come in and see her, she is alive!" there was a shockwave that hit them all. The crying stopped. Anger and fear began to come up from their souls in disbelief. They couldn't stand or walk but sat down. The nurse walked out with baby Sophie, "Is this yours?" she said. "We can't find anything wrong with her. I understand she was thought to be dead on arrival? Her eyes check out. She speaks and reflexes are working." Luke filled out his paperwork truthfully. "Child DOA, (dead-on-arrival) in ambulance a spontaneous revival occurred." This was the first of many such spontaneous revivals. The medical term for miraculous healing is "spontaneous recovery" Luke knew that. How was he going to get this raised-from-the-dead child past his peers and managers? The only hope he had was it will be ignored. Don't-ask-don't-tell will be the policy, he thought. As long as this hospital doesn't get on the news saying there was a child raised from the dead, everything is cool. If there is a claim of miraculous recovery, the hospital and his EMT company will be questioned and found ridiculous. Their credibility will become null or else he may be asked to change his documentation. No business wants to be accused of in-credulity. You can just about count on any medical establishment to have a circle with a line through it on the wall, "No Miracles Here." Miracles are just not welcome in medical establishments. Luke knew he had best keep it on the down-low so as not to cause sparks. He could feel the pressure already. One minister Luke learned about had actually raised his own adult son from the dead after 5 hours in the morgue. The hospital didn't tell the story or deny it, the minister says. It's predictable and biblical that unbelief will not be changed by way of miracles alone. Those who refuse will not believe even if someone is raised from the dead. (Luke 16:31)

Based on the testimony of Curry Blake (now of John G. Lake Ministries), raising his daughter from the dead. The daughter came back from death gasping as described "breathing in like she was thrown back into her body forcefully" after 45 minutes of standing on his faith declaring "she will live and not die."

The minister referenced here whose son was raised from death after 5 hours in a morgue is Andrew Wommack of Andrew Wommack Ministries in Colorado.

The missionary mentioned who often heals a deaf person on the spot to get attention and preach to a town was Heidi Baker, who is living somewhere in Mozambique, Africa.

Chapter 5

Here Goes Something!

Alex was a male nurse from an intensive care unit who had also been on the missions trip. He has been meeting with the team weekly, listening to testimonies and seriously struggling with the idea of praying on the job. Weeks have been passing and Barry has had opportunities but always slips into his medical knowledge. "After all I'm only human right?" he argued to himself today. The Holy Spirit inside of him answered in the voice of his favorite minister with a southern twang accent, "1/3 of you is wall-to-wall Holy Ghost!" Alex knew it was true. Conviction from the Holy Spirit is not condemning but it pokes and reminds us of our ability in Christ. He was being convicted of who he was in Christ, what his identity has been and is and what he has. Alex knew he could not keep being selfish with his ability to speak life over people. He could not hide his lamp under a bushel any more. What would he say in heaven when asked why he didn't use what he had in Christ on his job? What about the people who might live instead of dying? Alex knew he could be an Undercover Miracle Technician. Why would anyone do miracles undercover you ask? It sounds weak and seems like a cop-out but

actually, miracles under cover is biblical; Jesus did miracles undercover. He even told people not to tell anyone at times. He could not blow his cover because Jesus' secret mission on earth was to die for us. Jesus was the undercover Messiah. It was a surprise to Satan that Jesus was here to die. If the demons of this world had understood the mission they would not have promoted the crucifixion of the Lord of glory. (1 Corinthians2:8) So Jesus was an undercover Messiah and we can be undercover miracle technicians in order to do God's work. Alex imagined himself praying and commanding life over someone during work. His spirit was willing but his natural mind was weak. "How can I keep leaving my supernatural knowledge out of my career when that is where I need to be supernatural?" He thought to himself. "I agree. It's about time" came a thought from the Holy Spirit right after that. Peace flooded his previously tweaking mind. Relief came with that decision like air leaving an overfilled balloon. The Holy Spirit was ready and waiting to take action. Next day, sure enough, Alex had an opportunity. A man was admitted with a bloated belly. His liver was failing. Jaundice was evident and he was having trouble breathing. Alex and other nurses worked to intubate the man. Doctors swarmed him and his wife was instructed to get his affairs in order. This man was dying. Alex welled up with compassion and began praying "life!" he muttered. The man's wife was a Christian. She was talking on her cell phone asking people to pray for a miracle. She held her husband's hand. Alex went beyond his profession and asked her "Are you a Christian?" "Yes I am" she said. "I'm Grace" "Are you open to prayer Grace?" "Yes of course!" She said eagerly. Alex grabbed her hand and said "I am going to command this disease to leave like Jesus cursed the fig tree ok? I am going to speak life to his body and tell it to live in Jesus' Name. Ready?" "Ok!" She gulped excitedly. Then he spoke with authority, "I command death to leave and infection to die! Go! We bind Satan and say get behind us! We speak life over John! And we command his liver to renew! Liver you start functioning perfectly! Every cell in John's body be energized and full of life!" Alex paused, looked at John, looked at the woman who appeared excited and hopeful, and he continued, "No weapon formed against John shall prosper! God's grace covers all his sins, Jesus paid for his life in full, including any disease! We command John's blood to be clean and pure like Jesus' blood. Amen?" Alex said, glancing at Grace and her husband. "Amen!" she squeaked. John was unconscious. Alex instructed Grace to speak God's word constantly, saying "thank you Lord that my husband will live and not die." Say it hundreds of times. If you stop to rest, go back to it again. Don't plan for a funeral. Don't speak death. That would be like pouring gasoline on the seeds of life I'm planting. You must cast down imaginations of death and every lofty thing that exults itself against the knowledge of God and His promises to us, 2 Cor 10:5. Keep speaking life to keep your mind from thinking anything else." Alex explained. Grace was paying close attention. "Thank you so much! I've been asking God for help! My husband is not a believer!" she said tearfully. Alex replied with a smile, "well Jesus healed unbelievers too so that they may be saved! The only thing I warn is that you never speak death over him because death AND life are in the power of your tongue too. Do not give in to speaking words of death. Keep saying thank you Lord that John will live and not die."

John's parents came slinking in sadly asking about funeral plans. Grace refused to speak of those things and after they left she faithfully spoke life over John. Alex watched as he came in and out attending to John. Doctors surrounded his bed curiously and spoke of his demise. Alex kept watch and it encouraged Grace just by his presence. Before Alex's 12 hour shift was over John began stirring and trying to talk. His hands were waving to get the tube out of his throat! Nurses were running in and out, doctors stopped in tilting their heads and taking vitals. A sudden turn for the better was beginning. John was getting angry and insisting the tube come out. The order to remove the tube came. John spoke "water" and then motioned for a menu. "Soup?" he perked up and his impatience was a good sign of improvement. Grace kept looking at Alex and saying "praise God, John! God sent us just the right people to care for you!" John nodded. Alex knew this was a step in the right direction for himself and felt a pat on the back spiritually. Death and life are in the power of the tongue and no disease can stand up against the speaking of life from God's word. Relentless words of life are like laser beams killing off doubts. Hope arises and death must flee.

This account was from a miracle through our own hands, praying over a friend who was in serious condition. My husband Mark and myself prayed over him and instructed the wife. The instructions written here were per Norvel Hayes' account of a young woman praying over her dying husband. However, we used healing verses in addition to the instructions given here. Constant focus on life is the key instead of imaginations of death. Jesus raised a dead girl by speaking to her and His own focus was that "she is not dead but only sleeping." Matthew 9:24. He (Jesus) also refers to Lazarus as sleeping in John 11:11. This is the truth spiritually which overrides or trumps the physical truth.

Chapter 6

Why Undercover?

The team meeting was full of testimonies. Each one inspired more people to be bold enough to act in faith. "What if it's not working when you do pray?" Tom spoke out to ask his question. The room fell silent and excitement took a dive. "Speaking life and not death is always appropriate, never stop. You know it's the only way to see results in faith. Always take authority and don't judge by what your eyes see." Pastor Mark responded quickly to quash that doubting spirit. "Just step out in faith commanding life. Expect it right away; watch for it but rest in the fact that's it's working. Words of life are planting life seeds. Do not water the seeds of life we plant with the kerosene of doubt and death. Speak life and then thank God that it's done continuously." Tom nodded and awkwardly found his seat. "Tom you have seen plenty of miracles yourself." Pastor Mark said encouraging him. "Yes but I'm just not doing it at work." he confessed. "Well just think life and not death; sometimes all it takes is your subtle comments like 'you're going to be fine!' even before you find out the problem. "Seriously!" Pastor Mark looked around at the group. "I do that in faith even when it doesn't look good. It's a form of prayer to bless people saying they will be fine! And then I throw in "in Jesus name!'" he chuckled. "Try to understand that we are Undercover Miracle Technicians. Why?? Because we are bringing a spiritual flashlight into a natural realm which is dark. It's their territory. It's awkward. We don't want to freak people out on purpose yet the whole world groans for the 'Sons of God' (that's us) to take their rightful place of dominion back. In Romans 8:22 it says the whole of creation groans and travails for us, the sons of God, to take our dominion and set the planet right. Why aren't we taking dominion? Why don't we tell the weather what to do? Some of us do that regularly." he grinned and looked around knowingly. "But mankind can do this ever since Jesus redeemed us all! Everyone can command hurricanes to dissipate and the storms to be still. Whenever they do, however, most are so naturally minded, they can't believe it happened even if it does. Train yourself to tell things what to do. That is being Christ-like! We are made in His image, after all."

Chapter 7

Two Languages

Thinking spiritually instead of naturally minded is like having two languages. You know English without thinking, then you learn Spanish or French and you have to focus in order to speak it; but thinking in that language requires daily practice. If the team wanted to think with their spirit mind, which breeds life rather than their carnal or natural thinking, breeding death, they had to practice daily. Soon they realized their own health was a daily matter of how they believe. Now this was hitting closer to home. "It's like work, believing supernaturally!" somebody complained. "Nobody likes change." Pastor Mark explained. "Laboring to enter the restful peace of believing supernaturally is just like the effort needed to change a bad habit. Thinking naturally or medically and thinking supernaturally as well is just as possible as speaking two or more languages. To the medical world we must speak in medical terms; except miracles are not in that language are they?"

"Yes they are." Brandy spoke up both meekly and boldly. Miracles are recognized by doctors because they do happen often! Unexplainable recovery is called 'spontaneous.' If we use their language, there might be a chance that we could help them recognize God's presence at work." "Ooo that's good!" Pastor Mark exclaimed, pointing at her encouragingly and several others agreed. He continued, "If we present miracles as common and acceptable possibilities, people would be healed more often. The fact that miracles seem impossible causes people to have more faith in the disease than in recovery. This is why we don't see as many miracles in the U.S.A. as in third-world countries. We have our faith in natural solutions so strongly, spiritual faith is quashed."

"Absolutely correct." Joel joined in. "In desperate places we will believe for the miraculous. Our first order of business here needs to be faith. Let's say, FAITH FIRST, in other words." Everyone agreed to start thinking spiritually-minded first. It wasn't long before that opportunity came up.

Brandy was home when her 4 year old daughter Lilley was sucking on a hard candy. Her husband Ben was in the garage when Brandy heard Lilley wheezing in the kitchen. Lilley was turning blue, opening her mouth and not speaking; Ben walked in and saw the look of alarm on both faces. The room was frozen with fear as if in slow motion,

Ben spoke sharply "Lilley! What's wrong!"   Brandy was standing at the counter watching. Her thoughts went to Heimlich maneuver but her spirit rose up unexpectedly and she shouted and pointed authoritatively at her precious child "Come out!!" The piece of candy was ejected violently across the room before daddy could move. In a moment of shock, the fear left and the child sucked in a breath and then heaved out and in her breaths, color returning to her face. Daddy scooped her up into his hugging position. "Are you ok?" He turned to look at mom who was tearing up in relief. "Wow" she said when she could finally speak. Ben wondering what just happened stared at her and waited for her explanation. "I..I guess my faith rose up and took over!" Ben was having a hard time speaking his thoughts. "So ..you had more faith in speaking to it than me! I'm usually the faith guy and you usually go to the medical training during emergencies." "Ya I recently decided to try a 'Faith First' approach. But I was surprised at my boldness too!" Brandy admitted.

This story is taken from a true account which happened to my granddaughter Lilley. Her mother Bethany, really did command it out even though she is an R.N. in an emergency room in Detroit and might have used the Heimlich. Daddy really is usually faith first and medical later.

Chapter 8

Fighting Back

Pastor Mark had the next Faith-First opportunity. He was at home doing laundry and as he started up the steps began to feel chest pains. The classic symptoms started. He stopped and put the basket down on the step. His left arm was in pain now. Leaving the basket he finished up the steps. Setting foot into his bathroom he sat on the toilet to catch his breath. Visions of a hospital emergency room flashed through his mind. It was 10 pm and no one was around in his home. The family was relaxing or else asleep, he wasn't sure.

Visions of his own funeral were forthcoming now. "That's a lie! I shall not die but live" he replied to the vision. "I shall not die but live and declare the works of the Lord. Psalm 118:17" The chest pain subsided and his breathing became deeper. Fear attempted to attack him again "You'd better call 911! You're having a heart attack!" thoughts shouted at him in his head. "I'm not having a heart attack, Jesus paid it all! You lying symptoms can't fool me." Pastor Mark insisted. The chest pains came back in another wave. He started sweating, the left arm was shooting pain up to his chest and panic started again. He stood to his feet and started paying in tongues. "No weapon formed against me prospers!" Pastor Mark declared. "This is my heritage as a servant of the Lord!" He continued to use his own tongue as a sword against the attack, "My heart beats with the rhythm of life.." Visions of his death flooded his mind. His wife at his funeral, his children, his grandchildren, his parents. Anger rose up and a righteous-indignation of faith, "I'm not dying! And even if I did I'll be with Jesus! Shut up!" he wheezed. His replies to those visions were meant to shut the mouth of the destroyer, the liar himself, the devil. As soon as Pastor Mark finished his declarations the symptoms vanished. The grip of fear also left and his strength came back. He looked at the color returning to his face in the mirror. He walked out of the bathroom and praised God for the authority He gave us as believers.

Based on a true testimony by Mark Suszek.

Chapter 9

Walk Away

Ben, the husband of Brandy, father and family man was on the trip but hadn't been willing to pray on the job either. Opportunity is not lacking where Ben works as a firefighter/paramedic by day or by night, but on his days off he is an Emergency Miracle Technician. Somehow he knew there had to be a way to combine these two superheroes into one. His life as a Christian was faith practiced at home, but medical and natural thinking at work. His trip to Uganda with the rest of the crew, highlighted his life and brought him to a new level.

Now, as his wife Brandy said, to see things change he wanted to commit to faith-first thinking. Resisting sickness had been well understood because of the ministries he followed for years. Now there had to be no more waffling.

Today was an opportunity to practice faith-first. Sitting in his truck waiting for his son Hunter to get out of school, Ben found himself suddenly nauseous. Little Hunter stepped into the truck and Ben hurried home. Parking in the driveway, his son jumped out and Ben was surprised by his own body projectile vomiting across the truck all over the seat. Ben hurled liquids he didn't know he had. Running to the house, thinking about the cleanup job in his nice Ford F150 with white leather interior, Ben made it for the second round into the toilet. "Dad! What happened??" Hunter cried. Ben tried to comfort him, "It's ok! I'll be ok!" Little Hunter looked for his mom. Ben laid down on the floor rebuking the vomiting and the flu. He had an appointment at 7pm and it was now 3pm. "Lord what is wrong? Why isn't it leaving?" The next thought Ben had was a conversation.

"What are you doing on the floor?" Came a gentle thought not his own. "I've got chills and a fever, I can't move" he cuddled the blanket tighter. No response. Ben remembered several other victories he'd had before. These memories were the Holy Spirit reminding him of how to trigger the results that were already his. Ben decided, (key word here is decided) to act on his belief that he's already well. "1 Peter 2:24 says I'm healed" he reminded himself. He still felt sick but he had a new thought, "do what you think you can't do."

That's not logical. No, it's spiritual. Spiritual thinking will bring us life and peace. And feeling like he was raising a dead man, he forced himself up with his will to be well and started down the steps walking away from the bathroom and the bedrooms. One step, two steps, three steps WHOOSH! It was gone. Relief came, the fever left, nausea and all. Gone! As fast as it came, it left. "Whoa! That was cool!" Ben said so loudly and excitedly, his son and wife heard him. "Dad did you get healed?" His son knew the sound of his dad's voice after a sudden and "spontaneous recovery." And so it was; Ben had simply walked away from the flu symptoms decidedly, knowing God's will was for his well-being.

Based on true testimony from Mark Bostwick of Live Move Believe Ministries, Northville Michigan. This testimony has helped me see results many times.

Chapter 10

Tug of War

Experience is the most helpful part of faith. Even when you experience and see a miracle your natural mind will try to excuse it and talk you out of believing it. Once you've seen it many times, then faith becomes knowledge and you know the miracle is always right there for the taking. Other people's testimonies become realities for you as well. With a mountain of victories under his belt, Anthony was prepared for the disaster that can happen to anyone but rarely does. Anthony was close to someone who had been healed of MS and so he was familiar with fighting the symptoms. His brother was diagnosed as a child but with the belief in healing they were taught, his symptoms reversed in a year. Wheelchair and all, paralysis was reversed. Now, there was a pop quiz of what he learned from brother.

Driving on the winding roads of Virginia one cannot see the other side of any hill. Maneuvering those twisting mountainous roads is a skill and any distraction could be deadly. This simple invitation to a family reunion in Jamestown launched a road trip that was almost life-altering forever were it not for the knowledge of faith required because as is so often the case, people's lives are *destroyed for lack of knowledge.* Hosea 4:6

A rainy morning increases the likelihood that something could go wrong on a mountain. Ambulances and accidents along the way were enough to caution a slower speed. As careful as

Anthony was, still an odd thing happened. The hill ahead on their two-lane highway proved to be treacherous as an oncoming green Ford pickup came over the hill on his side of the road! To avoid a head-on collision, he grabbed the wheel tighter to steer around the truck but his small Escort fishtailed skidding out of control down a ravine where a tree, refusing to budge, his car.

The immediate pain in his neck caused him to black out. His sister Violet found her way out through a window. "Anthony!" She yelled, grabbing his limp hand. And praying immediately she began to speak to this mountain. "By the blood of Jesus" she declared "life, life, life!"

 Being pinned by the seatbelt, Anthony hung like a marionette which pressed on a broken clavicle. He wanted to pull himself away from the pain but could not lift his head and couldn't feel his legs.

The ambulance and rescue team was there in a very long 15 minutes. The jaws-of- life were used to open the car like a tin can. "You have a broken neck sir, for one thing" the paramedics said as they pulled him out after placing a cushioned brace around his neck. Anthony groaned as he knew what that meant. But faith-first was his new motto and his immediate reaction was healing. "Reverse-now-in Jesus name" he spoke as he went in and out of consciousness. Violet was praying in tongues, riding with him to King's Daughter's Hospital near the accident. The small town of Churchville was aware of the horrible incident and word spread to their small newspaper. The family waiting for their arrival was too far to do anything but cry as they heard of it. The reunion would be tainted forever. However the difference would be in the outcome by faith. Anthony's mind was clouded with morphine and yet he remembered to fight. Paralysis is a thing to be resisted and fought off. It tugs on a person and if you tug back you can win. If not you could fall into a pit which is hard to climb out. Anthony began to fight with his mind and engage his spirit. Transferred to University of Virginia Hospital, Anthony was told that if no sensation or movement began to return in three days, after swelling in the spinal cord is reduced, the paralysis was usually a permanent thing. He knew that God's word says "every tongue rising up against you in judgement you shall condemn, this is the heritage of the servants of the Lord" so he condemned that diagnoses. "In this case, it is not permanent. I am healing as we speak."

He fought off every thought, every vision of himself being in a wheelchair. No matter what the doctors said, he went with God's promises.

"You're in denial" he heard a thought trying to reason with him in his head. "*Absolutely! I'm in denial* of the plan of the enemy!" he rebuked the devil trying to cause him to relax his fight.

"I reject all this in the Name of Jesus!" He shouted inside and then "ouch!" he shouted out loud. The nurses and doctors looked at each other at the foot of his bed. "You felt that?! That's wonderful" and they kept poking "ouch!" Anthony said again with a smile. The healing of his broken neck was inevitable but the process in medical practice is gruesome. A halo vest with metal bars was screwed into his skull at 4 points to keep the neck in traction. Paralysis from the chest down is bad enough and to add not moving the neck to it is an experience no one should have to have. "Your spinal cord is bruised but not severed. So far it seems that you are a C-6 quadriplegic." The doctors explained his diagnosis. But Anthony was ready with his counter judgement. "It won't be that way long" Anthony declared. "I'll be recovering quickly. I have a great Physician and He says I'll have a full recovery." The doctors wrote down his response. They had meetings about his faith and how they should react to his beliefs.

Thankfully, Christian doctors were brought on the scene next. Anthony was understood after that and was then allowed to deal with his situation with the positivity he wanted. "It's ok to believe that you will recover but the doctors have to tell you what they see." One shared with him. "I understand" Anthony warned, "just let me do my thing too. It's my battle, I'm not giving in to this."

In a couple of days, feeling was returning, toes were wiggling, his fingers could grip. His diagnosis changed and the doctors' team was documenting furiously. Confusion is common to a hospital team whenever spontaneous recovery occurs. The plans were changing by the hour. The spinal cord unit was not able to predict what happened next. The normal procedures could not be followed and it was all good. It was God's hand and it was awesome.

In a week they removed the halo vest because Anthony's legs were moving and xrays showed his spinal cord was not swollen or bruised anymore. His bones in the spine were mended as if it never happened. The metal bars and halo vest were in the way of his recovery so they decided to remove it all. "Misdiagnosis," "misreading the X-rays," "inexperienced doctors." Any of these reasons were considerations for the documentation of Anthony's unexpected recovery. Anything except "miracle." Phantom paralysis? Is that a thing? It was not on the books yet but they were writing it down. Anthony was walking with a cane and ready to be discharged.

Then a discouraging thing woke him up at 3:22 am the day before going home. He felt unable to move again. All the paralysis came back. Was this a nightmare? He couldn't believe it but it was really happening. "Jesus!" He screamed in his mind. Then he envisioned a tug of war with demons on one side and a bright light on the other end. He was in the middle of the rope and he had it tied around him like a mummy. Breaking free from the tug of war was just a matter of resisting. Anthony started squirming and refusing the paralysis to have him back. Then like a limb that fell asleep, tingling and warmth moved from the middle of his body to his extremities. Movement returned and he was stronger than the day before. By 4am it was all like a bad dream and yet it really happened. "Resist the devil and he will flee" Anthony remembered. Questions flooded his mind. How? Why? What if? Yet he had peace. Discharged to go home the next day, Anthony heard a lyric of a song in his head as he left. "Death where is your sting?" from New Creation by Leeland.

This injury incident depicted the accident and injury of myself, Lynne Suszek in 1985 on my honeymoon three days after my first wedding. It resulting in a spinal cord injury which has sustained these 34 years. My lack of knowledge about faith at that time definitely allowed the injury to remain, however, I believe and have concluded that the key to my healing is in fighting it and not being passive. I owe my miraculous health and outstanding quality of life for all these years to God's promise that "according to your faith it will be done unto you." My ability to give birth to and raise my five healthy children in spite of the injury has been another wonderful result of receiving what I believed.

*The healing in this chapter tells how it could have been different based on testimonies of healing from paralysis of author Tony Myers not only being healed once of paralysis from ALS but 3 more times as described, back and forth. *Also based on a verbal testimony of healing paralysis from Malaria by a pastor Seun which occurred in Nigeria.

Chapter 11

According to Your Faith

"Back at the ranch" as they say, the team of Undercover Miracle Techs shared their stories and questions. Anthony's story was such a victory and yet there remained a question too. "Not to bring anyone down but we must be able to do better than recovery." Anthony stood up to make his point. "What about not having an accident at all? The miracle of avoiding any collision is the real goal isn't it" Pastor Mark responded, "Excellent point Anthony, yes it's divine health we want, not get-sick-or-injured-and –recover over and over. So what's missing?"

"Where are the angels when we need them?" Tom was quick with his questionnaire and Brandy was quick with an answer, "Psalm 103:20 says angels harken to the voice of His word. So if we speak God's word in faith or simply believe in faith for miraculous results things will be different. In Acts 28:5 Paul simply believed he would be unharmed by the snake that bit him and shook it off into the fire."

"According to your faith let it be done unto you, Jesus said in Matthew 9:29." Joel chimed in from the back. Anthony continued, "That's good! I don't ever want to have another collision and the fear of it is like calling it in. So changing my faith to never having a collision no matter what will be my next faith goal. I've heard of three testimonies where the cars were going to collide but by faith, they went right through each other. Like a time warp the molecules spread apart and there was a blurry second then they were on the other side looking back" Joel offered. "Now that's what I'm talkin about" and Anthony sat down in relief. From his seat he said "ok I can believe for that."

Pastor Mark stood up, "Yes this is very helpful. We can avoid sickness and injury and even collision if we believe for it."

"Oh yeah," Joel agreed, "The worse thing a person can do is shout 'we're all gonna die!' as the plane goes down!' Joel went on "What we believe in the seconds that precede an accident will influence the outcome. If you see a car about to hit you, by habit whatever is in your heart will come out of your mouth. I saw on YouTube about a plane going down in some other country and a pastor shouted 'Jesus!' The plane crashed but nobody died!"

According to Your Faith

"These are the kind of things we should be hearing at churches, y'all" a meek voice came from the back. Everyone turned their attention to the voice of a girls who rarely contributed but has been listening intently at the meetings. Baseball cap on her head, dressed like a girl from the streets, perhaps homeless, Skyler spoke up to make her point. "Why don't churches talk about this stuff? They waste our time with so much fluff but miracles are what people need to hear. People want to become familiar with the power we have in Christ which dwells in us, and how it works. They want to know what miracles look like. It's not just a rare occasional thing! It's a lifestyle for mature believers. In Hebrews 5 it says, (she read from the Bible)

[11] Of whom we have many things to say, and hard to be uttered, seeing ye are dull of hearing. [12] For when for the time ye ought to be teachers, ye have need that one teach you again which be

70

the first principles of the oracles of God; and are become such as have need of milk, and not of strong meat.[13] For every one that useth milk is unskilful in the word of righteousness: for he is a babe.[14] But strong meat belongeth to them that are of full age, even those who by reason of use have their senses exercised to discern both good and evil. "

"Amen" the room said in unison. Then Pastor Mark said, "We are an undercover-underground-miracle-technicians church. Bringing our faith to the world in spite of the church's immaturity is starting this way because this way, we can have more influence. The world rejects anything it doesn't understand. Provoking the world to jealousy and causing them to ask questions is actually scriptural."

> "...I magnify my ministry in order somehow to make my fellow (church members) jealous, and thus save some of them from deception."
> Romans 11:13-14   (Lynne Suszek Version)

The testimonies discussed about cars blurring through each other and ending up on the other side instead of collision was from Daniel Amstutz of Andrew Wommack Ministries and Tony Myers. It happened to both of them among others I've heard. Another one I heard from Andrew Wommack was about cows being in the road. (Yes, MOO cows)

*The Youtube plane crash discussed did happen. I found it myself.   Passanger shouts out in Jesus Name Plane Crash Miracle! 31 July 2018

www.ingramcontent.com/pod-product-compliance
Lightning Source LLC
Chambersburg PA
CBHW071230220526

45468CB00002B/796